Legal & Disclaimer

The information contained in this book is not designed to replace or take the place of any form of medication or professional medical advice. The information in this book has been provided for educational and entertainment purposes only.

The information contained in this book has been compiled from sources deemed reliable, and it is accurate to the best of the Author's knowledge. However, the Author cannot guarantee its accuracy and validity so cannot be held liable for any errors or omissions. Changes are periodically made to this book. You must consult your doctor or get professional medical advice before using any of the suggested remedies, techniques, or information in this book.

Upon using the information contained in this book, you agree to hold harmless the Author from and against any damages, costs and expenses, including any legal fees, potentially resulting from the application of any of the information provided by this guide. This disclaimer applies to any damages or injury caused by the use and application, whether directly or indirectly, of any advice or information presented, whether for breach of contract, tort, negligence, personal injury, criminal intent, or under any other cause of action.

You agree to accept all the risks of using the information presented inside this book. You need to consult a professional medical practitioner in order to ensure you are both able & healthy enough to participate in this program.

Contents

Introduction

With technological advancements, people are getting busy by working for the entire day to achieve great milestones. It is becoming quite difficult for people to strike a balance between personal and professional life. In such scenarios, maintaining a healthy lifestyle becomes quite challenging.

Cities are flooding with fast food outlets day by day. Consumption of such processed food can lead to long-term repercussions.

Right from the age of 30, you need to keep a check on the diet or food you are consuming. You just have to put in little effort and time in the right direction. Once all the things are done right, you could see some drastic changes within a small period.

Whenever we think about healthy food, there are a lot of doubts or questions that linger in our minds.

Some common questions that linger in the mind are:

- How much should a person consume in a day?

- What is BMI (Body Mass Index)?

- How many calories should a person eat in a day?

- What is considered to be a balanced diet?

These are some of the things that come to our mind when we are trying to work out a diet plan on having healthy food.

You need to understand what it means to have healthy food.

Chapter 1
Fundamentals of Healthy Food:
Elaborate the Benefits of Healthy Food with 10 Examples

What Do You Mean by Healthy Food?

Healthy food is generally considered to be something that provides essential nutrients to your body. A food that helps you to stay healthy, feel good and have an immense level of energy throughout the day. The nutrients that are available in healthy food are proteins, vitamins, carbohydrates, fats, and minerals. Eating healthy food and keeping yourself hydrated is the best way to keep yourself physically active.

Moreover, you would be introduced to the fundamentals of healthy eating which will have immense benefits on your body health. These benefits are the key to having the right diet which would keep you fit and healthy for a lifetime.

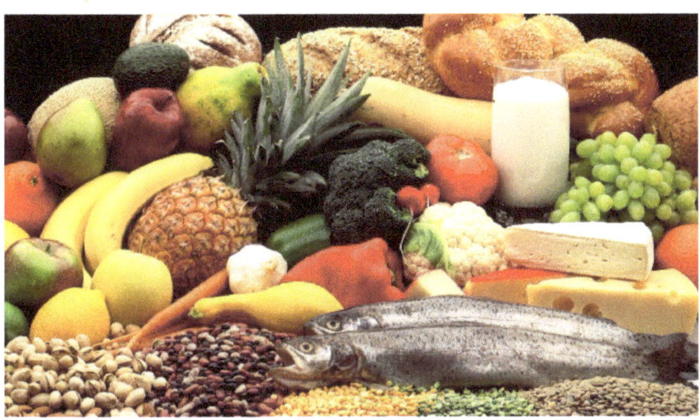

#1 You Must Know Yourself:

You might come across different kinds of people. For some, it would be a great pleasure to prepare your own food and for others, the microwave becomes a lifesaver. But the main thing here is to provide or learn a healthy way to cook and eat the food that work

For your body. A lot of online platforms would suggest going for several small meals rather than having everything in one go. But it depends on everyone's body structure and also their lifestyle. So, you need to be very wise while making a choice between the two. This point also suggests that you need to be aware of your pitfalls or limitations and try to avoid them.

#2 You Must Limit Yourself From Packaged Food:

You might have encountered many nutritionists who would recommend buying only fresh food from the supermarket. You must get hold of all the fresh food such as fruits and, vegetables, but avoid highly processed food. The trick here would be to turn a blind eye to all packaged food items. You also need to figure out if your food has essential elements such as fiber, potassium, calcium, and vitamins.

#3 Monitor Your Food Portions:

The best thing that you can do for yourself is to regularly monitor your food portions. The amount of food you are having in a day should have essential ingredients. People would also wish to have a cheat day when they could have meals of their choice. Moreover, there is a need to keep an eye on the number of calories that you would be consuming in a day.

#4 Always Segregate Your Fat:

This is the specific area of nutrition which is most confused. With this small tip, you would be able to know that fat provides more calories per gram as compared to other nutrients such as carbohydrates, and proteins. While maintaining body health, you need to monitor the amount of fat you consume in a day. Moreover, it would be beneficial to understand what impact it would have on your body. As per the research paper on "Health Effects of Polyunsaturated Fatty Acids in Seafoods" by The National Institutes of Health, Bethesda, Maryland, polyunsaturated and monounsaturated fats are considered good fats. These kinds of fats are found in vegetable oil, fish oil, salmon, trout and herring. These fats won't be adding any sort of cholesterol to the body. It is beneficial in reducing cardiovascular problems.

Now you might be wondering as to what can be included in the healthiest food. The given list provides foods that are both tasty as well as healthy. You can easily fill your plate with these fruits, vegetables, and quality protein. This would make an entirely versatile diet.

Fruits That You Need in Your Diet:

#1 Apple:

Fruit that is rich in fiber, vitamin C, and antioxidants. It can prove to be a perfect snack when you are hungry in between your meals.

#2 Avocado:

It is loaded with fat instead of carbs. It is very creamy and tasty and provides fiber, potassium and vitamin C.

#3 Banana:

It is the best source of potassium and is rich in vitamin B6 and fiber. It is very convenient as well as portable.

#4 Blueberries:

Fruit that is a powerful antioxidant and also very delicious.

#5 Orange:

It is a well-known source for Vitamin C. It is very high in fiber and antioxidants.

You can find various other fruits which are equally healthy. You can have mangoes, watermelon, black-green grapes, olives and peaches in your diet routine.

Poultry - Meat Products That You Need in Your Diet:

#1 Egg:

An egg is a powerhouse of various nutrients. It provides minerals, proteins, iron, and carotenoids. Eggs are considered to be the most nutritious food available today. They do not add any cholesterol to your body and are completely healthy.

#2 Meat:

Meat provides vitamin B, vitamin E, protein and magnesium.

#3 Chicken Breast:

Chicken Breast is rich in protein. Along with that, it is rich in vitamin B6.

#4 Lean Beef:

It is a highly nutritious food providing vitamin B6 and cobalamin.

#5 Lamb:

Lamb is a good source of protein, which is best for building strength.

Nuts & Seeds That You Need in Your Diet:

They are considered to be very high in calories but still the best source when you are seeking ways to lose weight. They are crunchy and loaded with all the important nutrients.

#1 Almonds:

These nuts are very rich in vitamin E, antioxidants, magnesium, and fiber.

#2 Chia Seeds:

With chia seeds, you get fiber, magnesium, manganese, calcium.

#3 Coconuts:

These are loaded with fiber and fatty acids called MCT - Medium-Chain Triglycerides.

#4 Walnuts:

Very nutritional nuts and high in fiber, vitamins, and minerals.

#5 Peanuts:

These are quite tasty and very high in nutrients and other antioxidants. These are the best ways to lose weight.

Vegetables That You Need In Your Diet:

#1 Asparagus:

A popular veggie, which is low in carb and rich in vitamin K.

#2 Bell Peppers:

You might be aware of the bell peppers (red, yellow, green). The best source of antioxidants and vitamin C.

#3 Broccoli:

It is an excellent source of C & K along with protein.

#4 Carrots:

A popular root vegetable. It is very crunchy which provides fiber and vitamin K and also high in antioxidants.

#5 Cauliflower:

One of the versatile vegetables. You can make a multitude of healthy dishes that taste good. It is rich in vitamin B6, vitamin K, and vitamin C.

Dairy Products That You Need in Your Diet:

#1 Yogurt:

Yogurt is considered to be highly nutritious and is an excellent source of protein, calcium, and potassium. It provides numerous vitamins and minerals and is relatively low in calories.

#2 Milk:

Milk provides several nutrients such as calcium, iodine, potassium, phosphorus, and vitamin B-12.

#3 Cheese:

Cheese contains a high amount of vitamin B 12, vitamin A and zinc.

#4 Butter:

Although we know that butter is high in calories but it also provides vitamin A, vitamin E and vitamin B-12.

#5 Buttermilk:

Buttermilk is considered to be a good source of calcium, vitamin D and protein.

Chapter 2
10 Quick And Easy Healthy Meal Recipes That You Can Cook

Here you will find some quick and healthy recipes which you can easily cook in your home.

#1 How to Prepare Broccoli | Tips to Cook Broccoli

Crispy Broccoli | Preparation Time: 15 minutes

Broccoli is often considered very boring, but the fact is, it needs to be cooked right. Broccoli is juicy, fresh, firm and nutrition rich.

This is a quick and crispy recipe that can be prepared within a few minutes. Dice broccoli into small pieces and layer it smoothly with olive oil and salt (to taste). Now let it get cooked in the oven. If you wish to be more creative with broccoli, then you can grill, sauté or bake the florets.

Once the broccoli is cooked let off steam and the florets will absorb the flavor and not get soggy.

Highlights

- First cultivated in Europe, Broccoli yields a very high nutritive value.
- It is a very versatile veggie and can be used to make a number of dishes.
- Broccoli also ranks as the world's fifth most popular vegetable

[Source: Wikipedia]

#2 How to Prepare Cauliflower | Tips to Cook Cauliflower

Warm Cauliflower and Dukkah Salad | Preparation Time: 20 minutes

This is the best cauliflower dish that you can prepare within minutes. It will provide you with a warm feeling that won't leave you hungry. You can cook the cauliflower with pistachio and olive oil. Initially, just roast the cauliflower florets in some olive oil, salt, and pepper. Once the florets turn into the golden-brown color you have to sauté it into the saucepan with some garlic paste and lemon juice.

When you have prepared this, you need to proceed with Dukkah. To make Dukkah, you will have to ground some pistachio, along with coriander, cumin, sesame, and chili. Finally, to make a salad you have to add some slices of nectarines, avocado, and mint.

#3 How to Prepare Bell Pepper | Tips to Cook Bell Pepper

Roasted Bell Pepper Salad with Mozzarella and Basil | Preparation Time: 15 minutes

Mostly, bell peppers are available in different types such as red, yellow, orange, and green. This recipe is a Caprese-style salad and it can be paired with some fresh mozzarella and acidic balsamic drizzle. You can also try some green bell pepper if you are not a great fan of sweet ones. This recipe could be prepared just within 20 minutes. In the process, you have to boil the bell pepper in a bowl and keep turning them. After 10 minutes, you need to check whether the bell peppers have become soft and tender. Finally, serve it with mozzarella cheese, basil, oil, balsamic glaze, salt, and pepper.

#3 How to Prepare Carrots | Tips to Cook Carrots

Moroccan Spiced Roasted Carrots | Preparation Time: 20 minutes

For this recipe, you will require some tender baby carrots. Just scrub the carrot and slice them evenly. In a bowl add sliced carrot, olive oil, ground cumin, paprika, ground cinnamon, and kosher salt. Toss them properly. Bake the mixture for 15 minutes. You can pair this roasted carrot with lamb or sometimes beef or curry as well.

#4 How to Prepare Asparagus | Tips to Cook Asparagus

Asparagus Turkey Stir-Fry | Preparation Time: 20 minutes

If you are looking for a wholesome healthy meal prepared from asparagus, then this is the best recipe you would ever find. It is delicious and also provides health benefits.

In a bowl, you need to add cornstarch, lemon juice, along with turkey and garlic paste. Mix it along with olive oil and bake it until the turkey becomes a slight golden-brown. Stir-fry asparagus in the left-over oil until it gets tender and crisp. Toss the mixture well and serve it with coriander

#5 How to Prepare Eggs | Tips to Cook Eggs
Loaded Scrambled Egg | Preparation Time: 15 minutes

We already know the benefits of eating eggs. Here is a quick recipe that will help you to prepare amazing eggs within a few minutes. You will need some eggs, a non-stick pan, olive oil, salt, and pepper. In the pan add olive oil, onion, bell pepper, salt (to taste), pepper and stir till they become tender. Add the eggs to the mixture along with cheddar, parsley, and tomatoes. Serve this recipe with tomato soup.

#6 How to Prepare Chicken Breast | Tips to Cook Chicken Breast

Lemon-Thyme Chicken with Sautéed Vegetables | Preparation Time: 20 minutes
This recipe will help you to gain energy and stay fit. As olive oil is used, it won't be adding cholesterol to your diet. In a bowl, you need to add some lemon juice, garlic, thyme, salt, black pepper. To this, you need to add chicken tenders. Now in a non-stick pan, you need to add some olive oil and pour the entire mixture to it along with a slice of zucchini ribbons. Let it cook for 15 minutes and then serve it with some mint leaves.

#7 How to Prepare Almonds | Tips to Cook Almonds

Chocolate-Almond Hearts | Preparation Time: 10 minutes

Almonds are good for skin and health. With this recipe, you will be using blanched almonds which are white nuts with no brown covering on it. They are easily available in the market. In the process, you will have to dip the almonds halfway into the bowl of melted chocolates by pointing them down. Now lay the almonds side by side, pointing towards each other and touching on a wax paper or butter paper. It will take the shape of a heart. Now let them stand until it gets firm or you can also freeze them. You can serve the almonds chilled.

#8 How to Prepare Walnuts | Tips to Cook Walnuts

Walnut Toffee Tart | Preparation Time: 17 to 18 minutes

Initially, in a bowl, you would have to add white flour, sugar, butter, egg yolks, and blend it properly. When the dough is ready, place it on the pan with butter paper. Now sprinkle the walnut onto the dough along with the melted chocolate. Now let the entire mixture to baking till 12 to 15 minutes at 375 degrees. Once this is done you can let it cool down and then serve it with tea or coffee.

#9 How to Prepare Apples | Tips to Cook Apples

Warm Cinnamon Apple | Preparation Time: 15 minutes

This is a simple spicy apple recipe that is perfect for any occasion. You can season it with an additional bowl of vanilla ice cream. For this recipe, you will have to dice the apple and put it in a bowl. Add some cinnamon, butter, ground nutmeg, brown sugar and water to it. Toss the mixture well and add it to the saucepan and stir it for about 8to 10 minutes until the apple becomes tender. Now serve it with some whipped cream as a topping.

#10 How to Prepare Bananas | Tips to Cook Bananas

Banana Oatmeal Pancakes | Preparation Time: 25 minutes

In this recipe, you have to prepare the batter for the pancakes and add some bananas and oatmeal along with walnut to it. Stir the mixture well. Now pour half cup batter onto the griddle and spray some cooking oil on it. Let it cook and turn it only when the bubbles start to form on the top of the pancake. You need to cook till the other side becomes golden brown. Your pancake is ready to be served. You can serve it with a glass of milk.

Chapter 3
Tips to Preparing Healthy Food to Optimize the Benefits to the Body

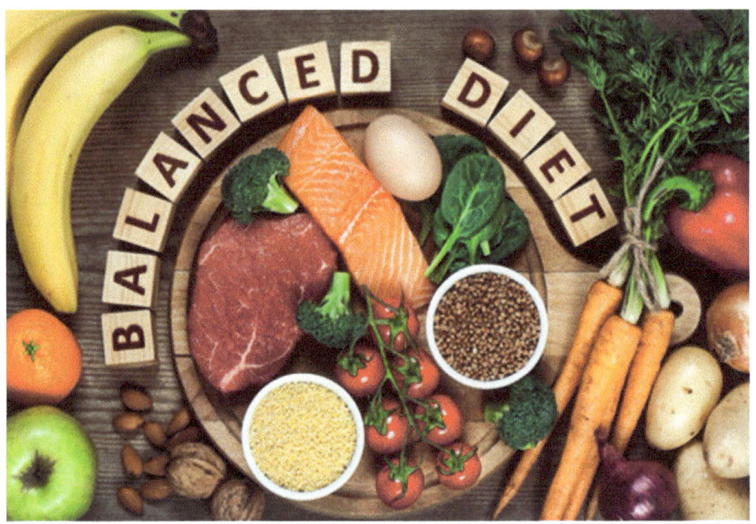

Healthy Eating! When these words ring in your mind you suddenly think that you need to cut down on your favorite food. But this is not so. Healthy eating does not necessarily mean that you need to give up your favorite food. There are numerous alternative ways in which you can adapt your favorite recipes to provide healthier options. For instance, you can opt to have non-stick cookware so that you can reduce the use of cooking oil. Another way would be to steam or microwave the vegetables instead of boiling them. When you boil your vegetables, all the valued nutrients are reduced.

Let's check out some more healthy cooking tips which can help you optimize the benefits to the body:

- Monitor the amount of fat, sugar, and salt added to the food

- Increase the consumption of vegetables, fruits, whole-grains, lean meat, and low-fat dairy.

#1 Low Consumption of Fat:

Make use of nuts, seeds, fish, soy, olives, avocado and limit the use of processed food which has hidden fat included. Even while cooking food you can make use of virgin oil or monounsaturated oils (olive oils or canola oil) that have low fat. They have long-chain fatty acids with good nutrition.

#2 Retaining Nutrients:

We are aware of the fact that water-soluble vitamins are quite delicate and can be easily destroyed while you are cooking food. So, to minimize the nutrition loss:

- Try to scrub the vegetables instead of peeling them off. This is said because many nutrients are found close to the skin of the vegetables.

- Instead of boiling the vegetables, try to steam or microwave them. (If you prefer to boil them make sure that you are not overboiling).

- Opt to have stir-fry recipes in your diet. Stir-fried vegetables retain their crunch while cooking.

#3 You Must Cut Down on Salt:

Salt is something you cannot do without. It is the most common flavor enhancer. Most experts have suggested that having a high amount of salt in your diet can contribute to a wide range of health problems, which can include high blood pressure.

One small tip that you need to follow here is not to automatically add salt to your food. (You need to taste it first).

Some more healthy cooking tips:

- With a splash of olive oil, vinegar or lemon juice. It is the end of the cooking time or cooked vegetables. It will be helping you to enhance the flavors just like salt.

- Choose to have fresh vegetables as canned food has salt already added to it.

- Avoid consumption of any sort of salty food which is processed meat such as salami, ham, corned beef, bacon, smoked salmon and much more.

- You must always use iodized salt while cooking food.

- Choose to have butter and cheese that have added salt in it.

- Reduce the use of soy sauce, processed sauce and condiments as it contains a high level of salt.

Chapter 4
Best Practices to Stay Healthy with a Balanced Combination of Diet and Exercise

A phase comes in our lives when we consult our medical experts who always recommend us to have a combination of diet and fitness to gain good health. You must be wise enough to choose nutritious food. Along with that, you should workout regularly to maintain your overall health. It is very essential to have a combined thing and it is also proved by the American Heart Association. They state that having a combination of proper diet along with exercise is the best way to prevent yourself from diseases.

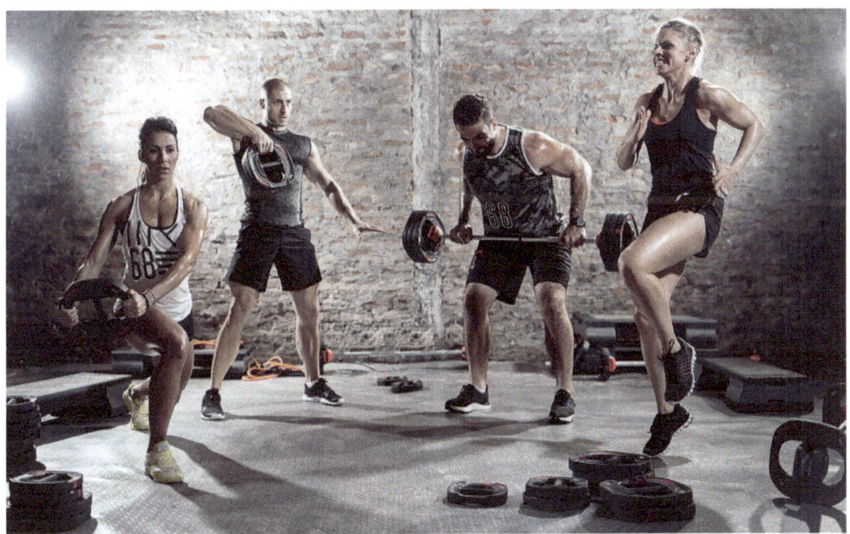

In the fast paced world, staying healthy has topped the list for nearly everyone's priority and it is helping them to determine how healthy they are.

Staying healthy is something that will keep you active in the long run. Our daily choices can determine just how healthy we are. Not everything is in our control, but the habits and approaches we take to our health can often make a difference between being healthy and unhealthy.

The two areas in which we have the most control over are our diet and exercise. These can both have huge effects on overall health and can be some of the main factors in preventing disease and other complications later in life. Preventive healthcare measures like proper diet and exercise can also help your budget.

What are some of the key benefits associated with a good diet and proper exercise? Let's look at that, but first, let's start with some general diet and exercise recommendations.

Let's look at some of the advantages of having a combination of a balanced diet and fitness to the body.

As per the International Dietary Guidelines, it is suggested that having a combination of a balanced diet and exercise would help you achieve optimal health. It is a very simple formula that has been around for more than a decade. The quotation goes as "Healthy Diet + Regular Workout = Healthy Mind & Body".

The main reason is when you consume proper food and do regular exercise, your body would be functioning well, and it will be receiving all the nutrients which are needed for the body to thrive and remain active throughout the day. Moreover, your workouts will improve body strength, endurance and body composition along with cardiovascular health.

Advantages of Combined Diet Plan and Workout:

- This combination would provide the body with the ability to achieve or maintain healthy body weight.

- It would impart a thinner appearance along with better muscle tone.

- It will increase the vigor and energy of the body.

- You would be experiencing a reduction in the risk of chronic diseases which generally include hypertension, heart diseases, diabetes, or undetectable cancer.

- It will aim to improve insulin sensitivity and help you prevent any sort of weight gain or metabolic issues.

- Your blood lipid profile would be improved which includes cholesterol and triglycerides.

- Your immunity would be enhanced.

- You would be experiencing better sleep

- There would be a reduction in stress.

Food	Eat With This Food	Do Not Eat With This Food
Protein-rich food such as meat, fish	Leafy green vegetables such as lettuce, spinach	Sugar or starched-filled food such as bread, pasta, crackers, etc.
Starches and Grains	Green salad, vegetables	Protein-rich foods and fruit
Melon	Do not eat with any other foods; always eat alone	Eat melon by itself
Vegetables (all types	Protein, starches/grains	Melons
Fruit	Okay to eat with most other fruits	Do not combine with other foods

Let's learn about the diet and workout synergy and how it will create an impact on the human body.

Diet and Exercise Synergy

For many years, we have been consulting our nutrition expert and they have been recommending it for monitoring the calories for proper weight loss and also to maintain it. Most of the experts have been recommending striking a balance between the intake of calories and the number of calories you are burning out.

Your body gets the calories from the food you have in a day. It is measured in the units of energy. A simple notion behind gaining more weight is to consume more calories as compared to the amount of workout you are doing. In addition to that, you can do regular exercise or some activities which would be helping you to spend your energy so that you do not gain much weight. Moreover, proper exercising will help you in the body's metabolic process and helps you to stay fit and healthy.

According to the studies, everyone who is seeking to maintain good health must strike a balance between proper diet and workout. One must try to avoid overcompensation of exercising by having an extra amount of food.

Definition Of A Healthy Diet

Let's check what do we mean by a healthy diet?

People these days are munching on the fast food just to save some time. But when it comes to body health, consuming fast food must be out of your list. Some people try to get healthy food during lunch or dinner. But what do you mean by having a healthy diet? Generally, a healthy diet comprises of:

- Your plate must have some whole grains, nuts, legumes.

- You must have a variety of fruits and vegetables at regular intervals.

- Daily get a small amount of lean protein and low-fat dairy products.

- An adequate amount of sugar (avoid using processed sugar), oil (use only the monounsaturated and polyunsaturated oils)

- Water is something that would keep you hydrated and active all day long. Make sure to have enough of it. (It can be consumed in the form of juices, smoothies, or health drinks.

-

 Try to avoid items just like bread and, fries. Water is something that will keep you hydrated and active all day long. Make sure to have enough of it. (It can be consumed in the form of juices, smoothies, or health drinks.)

Let's move ahead to check how to define fitness and what it means to stay healthy.

Do you think that hitting the gym once a day can help you stay fit? Or you can just do aerobics and yoga to maintain your health?

To achieve fitness, you need to concentrate on achieving all five major components of physical fitness. These components comprise of :

- Muscular Strength & Endurance

- Cardiovascular endurance

- Healthy Body Composition

- Flexibility - Yoga & Aerobics

- Good Food

You must have an effective plan that would help you in making the balance between all the above activities. There are some benefits to these activities and the effective plan as well.

- With the help of aerobics which you would be doing 30 minutes every day, you would be able to get desired results in a few months.

- If you are more inclined towards the strength training activities, then you need to work on the major muscle group - thigh muscles, abdominal muscles, and biceps. Try to work on it three times a week.

- Stretching is a must. It imparts flexibility to your body.

So the most important thing here would be to focus on having a goal to obtain good health. Having good health does not necessarily mean that you have to lose weight and get thin. By good health, we mean that you must know about your body requirements and then chalk out a perfect diet and workout plan accordingly.

Here we would be discussing some of the tips and tricks that would help you to strike a perfect balance between healthy living and proper eating.

How to Strike a Balance Between Healthy Food and Workout

- Working out on a regular basis is a must. If you are a beginner, then start from simple exercises like walking or jogging.

- Your good food and exercise will be supporting you to stay healthy all day long.

- Make a combination of moderate-intensity exercises and vigorous-intensity exercises.

- Try to work on muscle strengthening exercises twice a week.

- Adequate water consumption is very important to keep yourself hydrated.

Chapter 5
10 Exercises to Keep You Healthy

We are all aware of the fact that regular exercise is the best way to optimize your health. With that, you are also aware of the unlimited options that are available in today's time. But the essential point that you need to notice here is what exercise would work for you. But you need not worry, we bring you some of the greatest sets of exercise which would help you to stay fit and healthy for a long period.

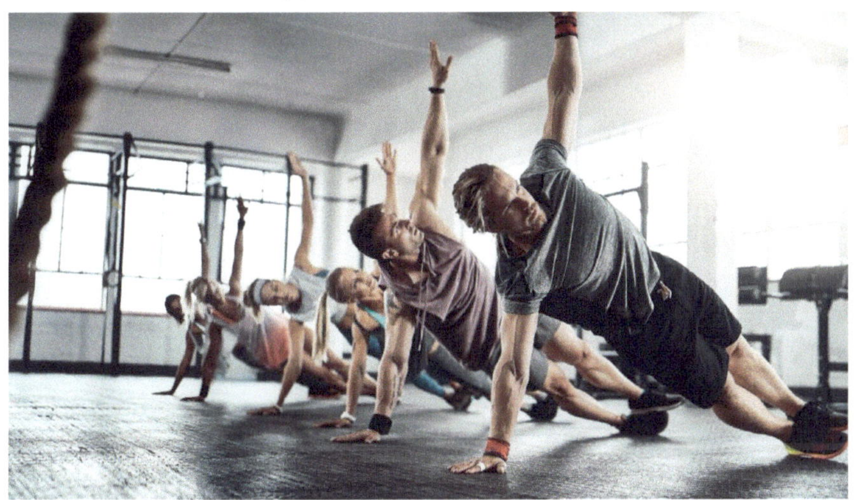

You can check out these 10 exercises to get the ultimate fitness and a perfect form. You can combine these exercises into your daily workout schedule. With this, you could keep yourself healthy, powerful and in perfect shape. Within a month, you could see improvements in muscular strength, endurance, and balance.

#1 Interval Training:

In the entire set of exercises, every exercise has a variable pace. In some exercises, you need to work out at a faster pace and in others, you can be a bit slow. For instance, you can do the walking exercise at a faster pace and push-ups at slower pace. By proper interval training, you can help your body to improve its regulations which include regulated heart rate, breathing, and metabolism.

All these exercises that we would be discussing help you to burn your calories, lose weight and also strengthen your muscles.

The essential thing is to maintain the intensity of your workout.

#2 Walking Exercise:

You must walk as it is one of the simplest exercises and yet very powerful. The aim is to help you stay trim, improve on your cholesterol levels of the body, strengthen the bones, monitor the blood pressure and keep a check on it. Moreover, it helps to lift your mood and focus to lower the risk of several diseases.

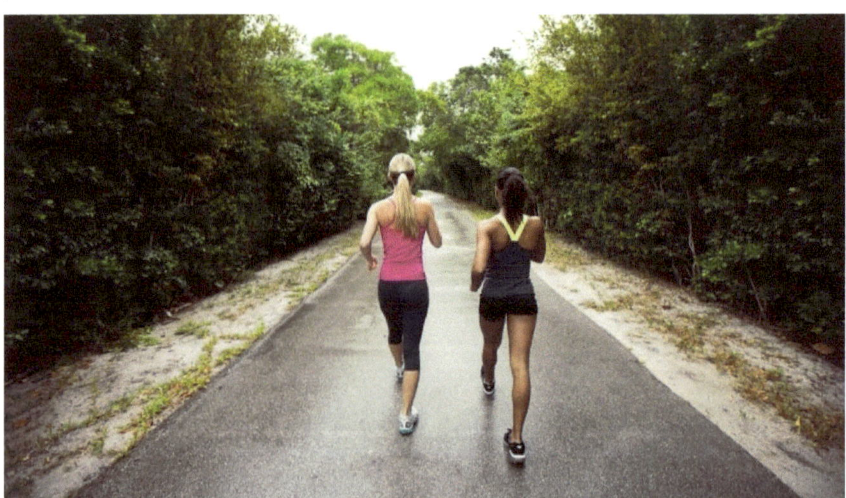

Numerous studies have shown that walking can help you to improve your memory and it will resist-age related issues. All that you need to do here is to get a pair of well-supported or well-fitting shoes and start your walking. Initially, you can start it for about 10-15 minutes and then gradually increase it to 30 minutes and then 60 minutes.

#3 Swimming:

You can consider it as one of the best or perfect workouts. Why is it called so? You can see that that the water in the pool has buoyance which is beneficial in supporting the body and then take away all the strain off the joints. It will help you to move with more fluidly. With various research and analysis, it was proved that swimming is also good for your mental health and helps to improve your mood.

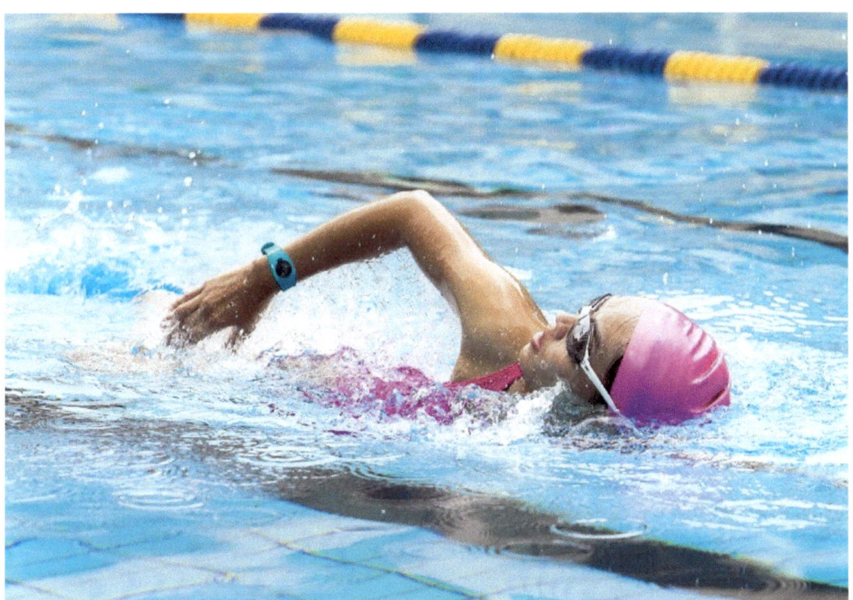

If you do not find swimming comfortable then try out water aerobics, which is another great option. It will help to tone up your body and burn the extra calories.

#3 Squats:

This one is just perfect for calorie burning. You must be wondering as to all the exercises that are aiming to do that! But in squats, your body's largest muscles are used. In this exercise, your body moves in the up and down motion. (It resembles the motion of getting out of the chair and sitting on it). The proper way to do the exercise is to keep your back straight, your feet must spread apart, both arms must be extended to the shoulder level. While your body is moving downwards make sure that your knees are over your ankles. It is recommended by most of the fitness experts to incorporate squats into your routine exercises.

#4 Working On Push-Ups:

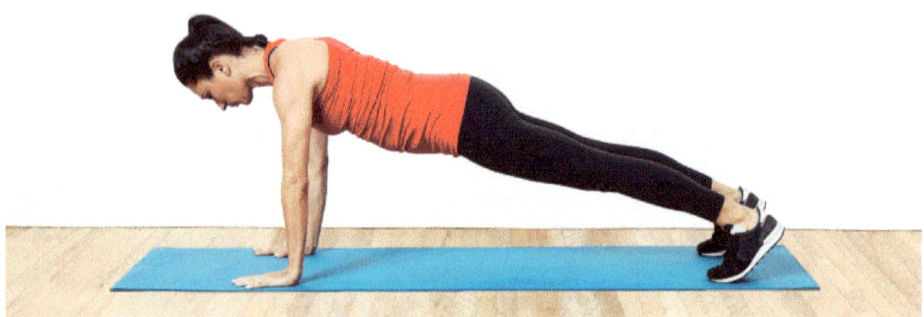

It is a classic exercise that helps to strengthen up the upper body (chest, shoulders, and triceps) and the core of the body (abdominal). If you are a beginner, start by spreading your legs apart, arms to the shoulder level and put it against some hard and unmovable object. Slowly bend down your elbows and go down till your chest touches the surface of the object. Ensure that you just have to allow your toes to bend and not the knees. To get a perfect form you need to keep your back straight.

#5 Working with Lunges:

Similar to the squats, lunges make use of your thigh muscles. With this exercise, you can improve your legs and enhance your balancing. The procedure goes by taking a big step in the forward direction and form a 90-degree angle with the knees.

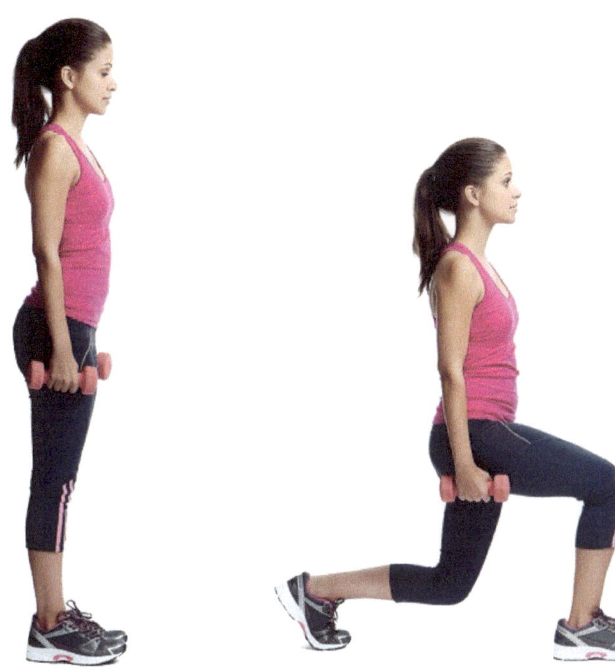

While doing the exercise you must keep your spine straight (no bending). The second leg would be trailing simultaneously and coming close to the floor. In this position, your toes would be experiencing significant body weight. When you are done with the first step you can repeat the same with another leg. If you are a beginner, then start with small steps and gradually keep increasing the placing between the legs.

#6 Crunches:

The best crunches exercise that you can do is the standard abdominal crunch. It has proved to one of the excellent ways to strengthen and shape the abdominal muscles.

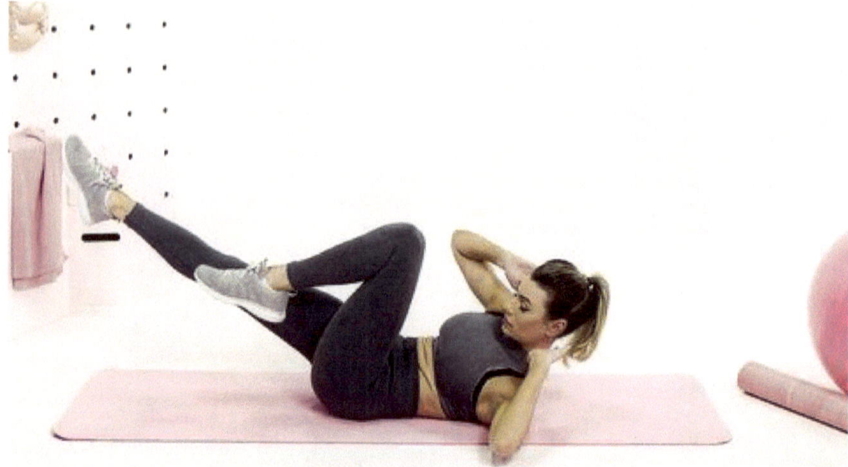

You would find it amazing to know that there are two different ways to start with this exercise.

#1 In the first one, you will have to lay down on your back with your foot flat on the floor. Keep your palms under your head. Now try to press your lower back down. In this process, your abdominal muscles (abs) will contract. Slowly raise your head, then neck, then shoulders and finally your upper back off the floor. Try to tuck-in your chin while bending forward. Now, lower your back down and repeat it several times.

#2 The second way is more interesting. In this process, you would have to do the crunches with your feet by lifting them off the floor and bending your knees. With this, you would not have to arch your back. Your legs will use hip flexors.

Note: To be an expert in crunches: Keep your neck in line with your spine, tuck the chin in, breathe deeply and keep the shoulders out of your line of vision.

#7 Working With Planks:

With this exercise, you would be able to focus on the deepest core muscles. It is a very static exercise in which you have to use your arms to raise your body off the floor and to maintain or hold the position for some time. Now if you are a beginner, then start with 10 seconds and gradually keep increasing the time by 30 seconds to 60 seconds. The best part of this exercise is that it can be done anywhere. You do not require any sort of equipment for it. Moreover, it would be just a few minutes of your daily routine to show some mind-blowing results.

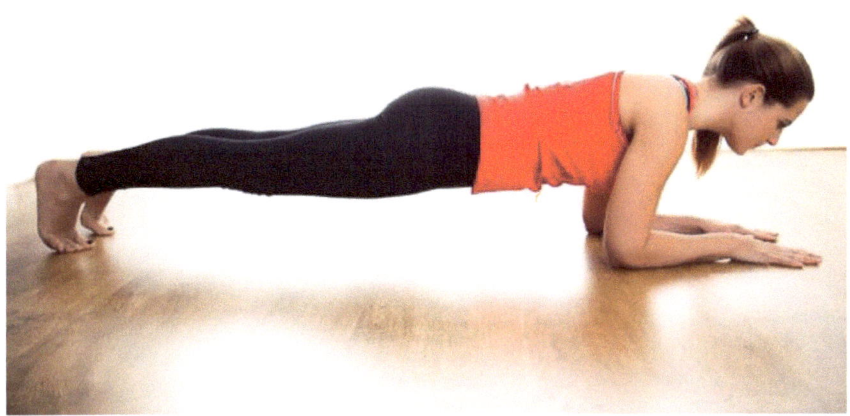

There are three different types of plank that you can perform alternatively.

Basic Plank: You can start with elbows and knees and lock your hands together. In the process, you have to straighten the legs and then raise your body and support it on the balls of your feet. You need to go just feet hip-distance apart. Now, face the floor and make sure that you maintain a straight back. Now hold this position for a few seconds. After doing it for once and twice you can gradually increase the time.

Side Plank: In the Side Plank exercise, you need to lie down on our right side/ left side and make your body propped up on your elbow. Make sure that your left foot is resting on the top of your right. Slightly keep pushing up your body. In this position, your body would be forming a perfect triangle with the floor. You must keep a check on your form as it must not roll down your shoulder. You need to hold the position as long as it is possible for you.

Prone Sky-Dive: Before doing this exercise you need to work on the basic and side plank. In this exercise, you need to lie down flat on the floor and your face down with your arms on the side. Now slightly raise your chest off the floor until you feel your lower back working. Make sure that you are not clenching your buttocks and try to hold the position for 30 seconds or more.

#8 Bent-Over Row:

In this exercise, you need to give proper exercise to the back and bicep muscles. If you are a beginner then stand with your feet shoulder-length apart and keeping your knees bent, hips should be flexed forward at the hip level. Now tilt your pelvis in such a way that it will contract your abdominal muscles. Do not extend the upper back and hold the position for a few seconds.

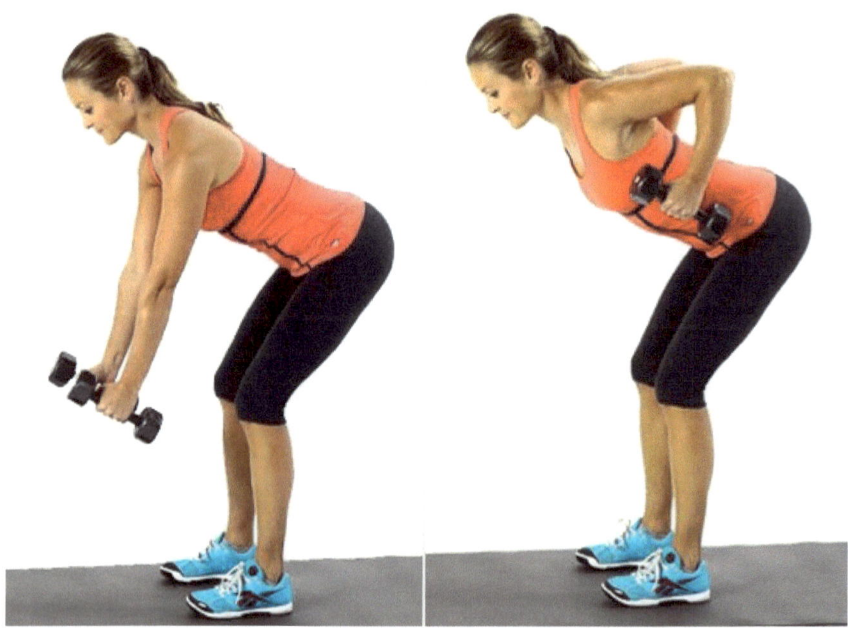

Once you are comfortable in your position, you need to flex your elbows in such a way that your forearms and hands move all way up. And repeat it again and again.

#9 Yoga:

Everyone is aware of yoga and the benefits that come with it. It will help you to increase awareness of your body posture, alignment and the patterns of movement. With yoga, you can be very flexible and help your body to relax even in stressful situations. This is the basic reason behind the increasing popularity of yoga. It will make you feel better, fit and also you would feel energetic throughout the day.

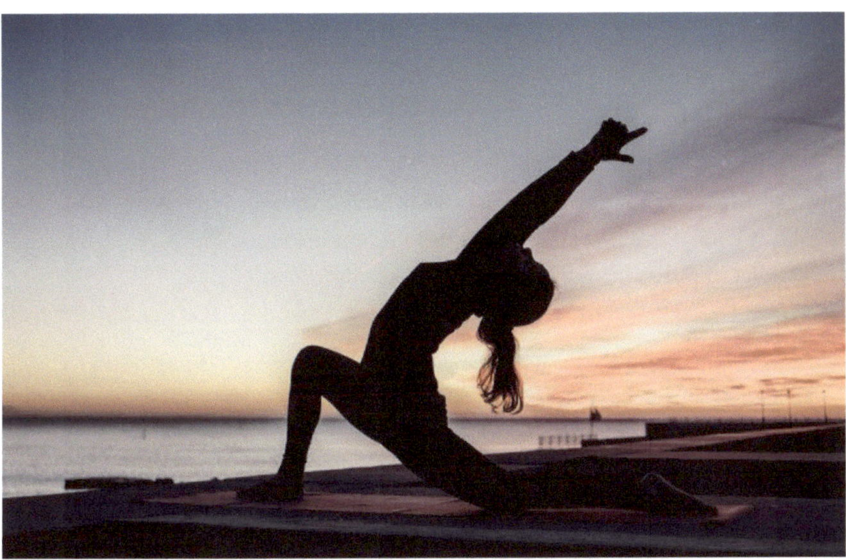

#10 Aerobics:

In aerobics, you will be giving motion to the entire body. The movement would be very fast which would raise your heart rate and makes you breathe harder.

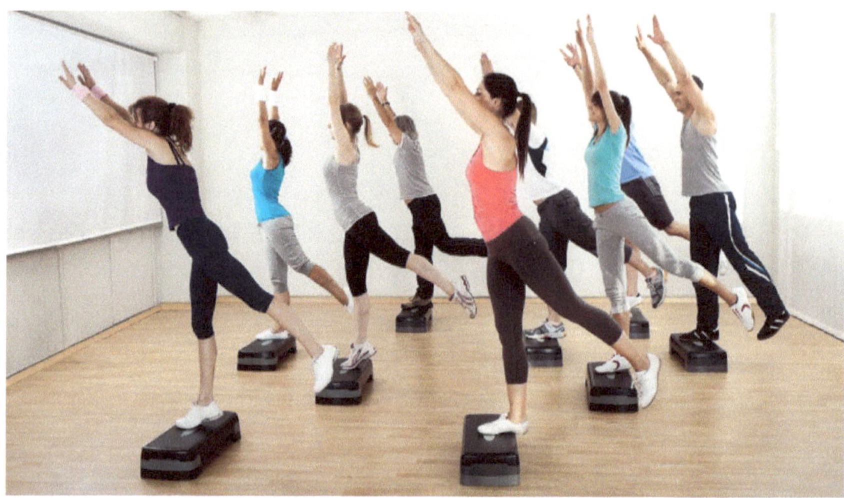

Final Note

It is very important to have the knowledge or to know about your health. You must be healthy enough before you try to engage in these activities. Moreover, consume a healthy diet to provide enough energy to your body.

Chapter 6
The Impact of Stress on our Body and How to Combat it

Are you feeling stressed out? The busy lifestyle of people is taking a toll on the personal as well as the professional life of every individual. It is the daily stress that builds up and has the potential to have a lasting impact on a person's health and well-being.

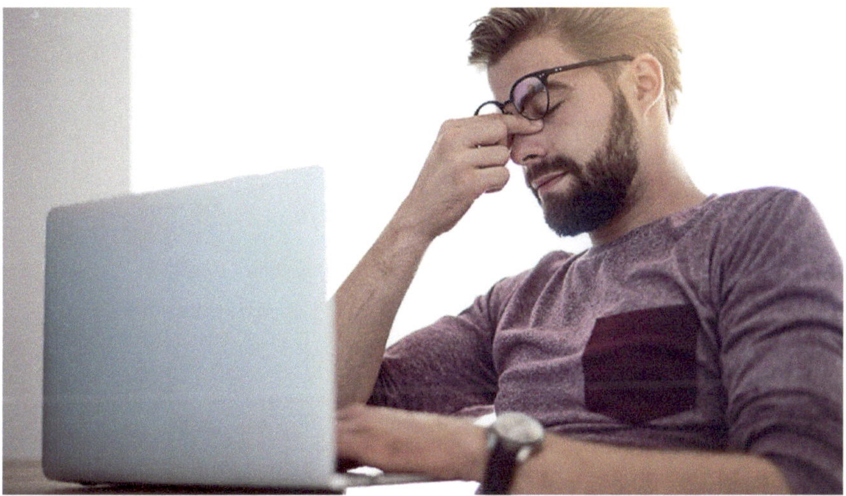

Stress has become an inevitable part of life, and every year we get to see the number increasing. In the analytic report of 2018, we were astonished to see that 80 % of people are experiencing at least one of the symptoms of stress. Stress can be due to positive as well as negative things. For instance, you can stress over an upcoming wedding or a new job or dinner date and other times it can be due to workload, family issues or health issues.

Stress is a thing that can affect you mentally as well as physically. Being under a stressful situation for a long time may put you at risk for health troubles like

- Digestive tract problems

- Anxiety

- Headaches

- Depression

- Sleep Problems

- Weight gain

- Memory and Concentration Issues

- High blood pressure

- Heart diseases or Stroke

So here comes the point as to how well you manage your stress and overcome it easily. You can always make some small changes in your life which are easy to try. It will help you to get a nifty life.

#1 You Must Giggle:

Try to spend some happy time with your family, friends or colleagues. To achieve that you can watch some funny videos of babies and puppies and any other thing that makes your belly moving. You can even try blowing some steam.

#2 Always Have a List:

When you make a list of things that are a priority to you then you can spend your next day without any stress. You would already be knowing what are all the important things or tasks that you need to complete. The bonus point here would be that you will have a sense of accomplishment when things are done properly.

#3 Find New Friends:

You can always take some breaks in your day to day activities to talk to your friends or meet them. You can also message them through social media networking sites.

#4 Travel:

This is a very general term, which does not necessarily mean that you need to travel to some exotic places only. You can go on weekend breaks or trekking or camping nights. It will help you to experience a lot of things and also make you feel stress-free.

#5 Dance and Music:

The slight movement of your body on the soft music can easily help you to relax your mind. It will give you a feeling that you are refreshing yourself by removing all the junk. You can try various dance-like hula whopping, brisk walking in the lane, hip hop.

#6 Proper Sleep:

Proper sleep will help you to stay productive and creative the next day. It has been recommended by the experts that you need to get to bed early and have about 7 to 8 hours of sleep a night.

#7 Meditation:

Meditation is something that will help you to focus or concentrate on your work and it will help trigger your body's relaxation response. Try to take deep breathes while you are meditating. It will enhance the impact of meditation and imbibe mindfulness.

Chapter 7
Various Health Benefits of Organic Food on Our Health

To strike a balance between our hard-pressed lifestyle and work, it is very essential to consume food that improves your health and helps you to stay fit. Now here comes the role of organic food.

What Do You Mean by Organic Food?

Basically, the term organic refers to the way agricultural products were grown and processed. So organic food is referring to the food products that are produced, prepared and processed without making use of any sort of chemicals, pesticides, fertilizers or preservatives.

Organic foods are becoming extremely popular due to the health benefits they are providing. It is good to have organic food as compared to the conventional ones. People have started realizing the importance or significance of organic food to improve their overall health.

Here are some advantages of consuming organic food.

No Harmful Chemicals:

Organic food does not contain any sort of chemicals, pesticides or synthetic material which harms to food or the soil. So it does not have any residual remains of the harmful chemicals.

Fresh Products:

Organic food is quite fresh and they do not contain any preservatives which make them last longer. Organic food is available from the small farmlands and it is not adulterated with any sort of chemicals.

Environment Safety:

As there is no use of harmful chemicals, it helps in reducing pollution, conserve water, reduce topsoil erosion, and maintains soil fertility.

No GMO/ GMO-Free:

Genetically Modified Organisms (GMO). Organic food is not genetically modified or genetically engineered.

Best For Overall Health:

It is quite easy to understand that organic food is not processed by the use of any harmful chemicals or pesticides. Hence, they do not contain any toxic elements which can prove to be harmful to the body. Organic food preparation makes use of natural techniques in which they use green pasture or manure to fertilize the soil.

Antioxidant Content:

Organic food is very rich in antioxidants and provides essential minerals vitamins that are required for the body. It limits your exposure to any sort of heavy metals.

Antibiotic-Resistant:

Humans, as well as animals, are susceptible to several health issues and here comes the role of organic food which boosts your immune system and helps you to stay healthy.

Conclusion

You must remember that organic food is always healthy. You should consume organic food and try to avoid junk food which might be delicious but not good for your health. So be careful and stay healthy!

–Justin Wheeler